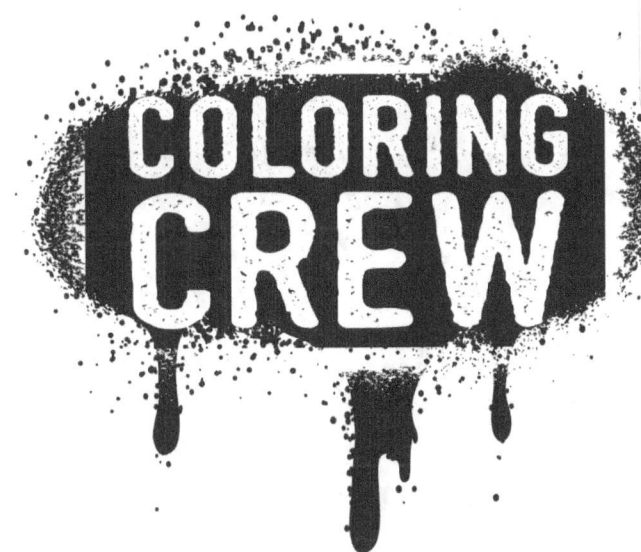

DO YOU SOMETIMES NEED TO SWEAR BUT CAN'T?

DOES IT ANNOY THE SHITAKE MUSHROOM OUT OF YOU?

WELL THEN THIS BOOK IS PERFECT!

EACH PAGE IN THIS BOOK HAS A RELAXING MANDALA CONTAINING A CLEAN SWEAR WORD THAT YOU CAN USE AS OFTEN AS YOU LIKE!

HAPPY COLORING!

Copyright © 2018 Coloring Crew.
All rights reserved.
ISBN-13: 978-1986928540
ISBN-10: 1986928543

COLORING CREW

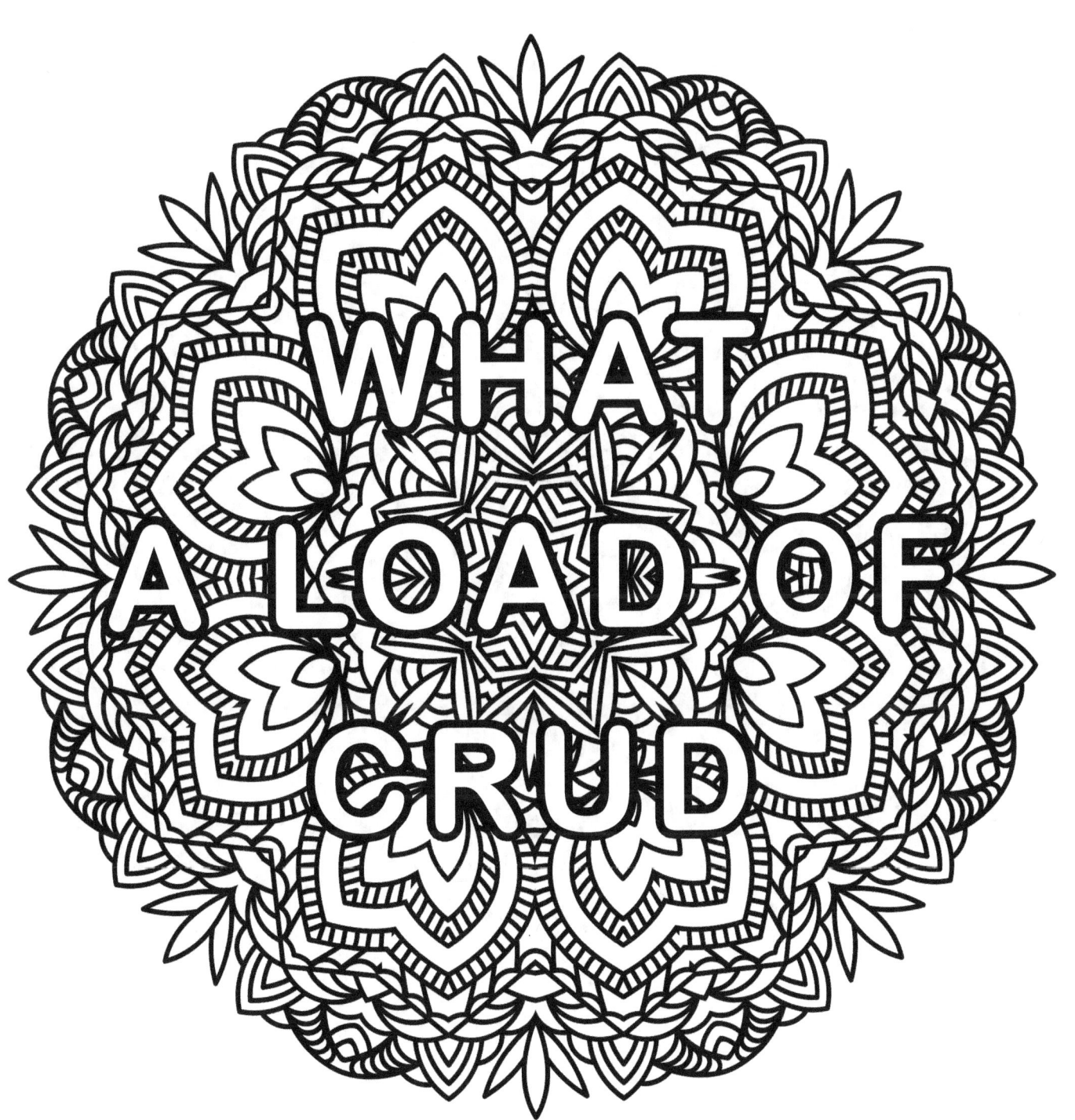

COLORING CREW

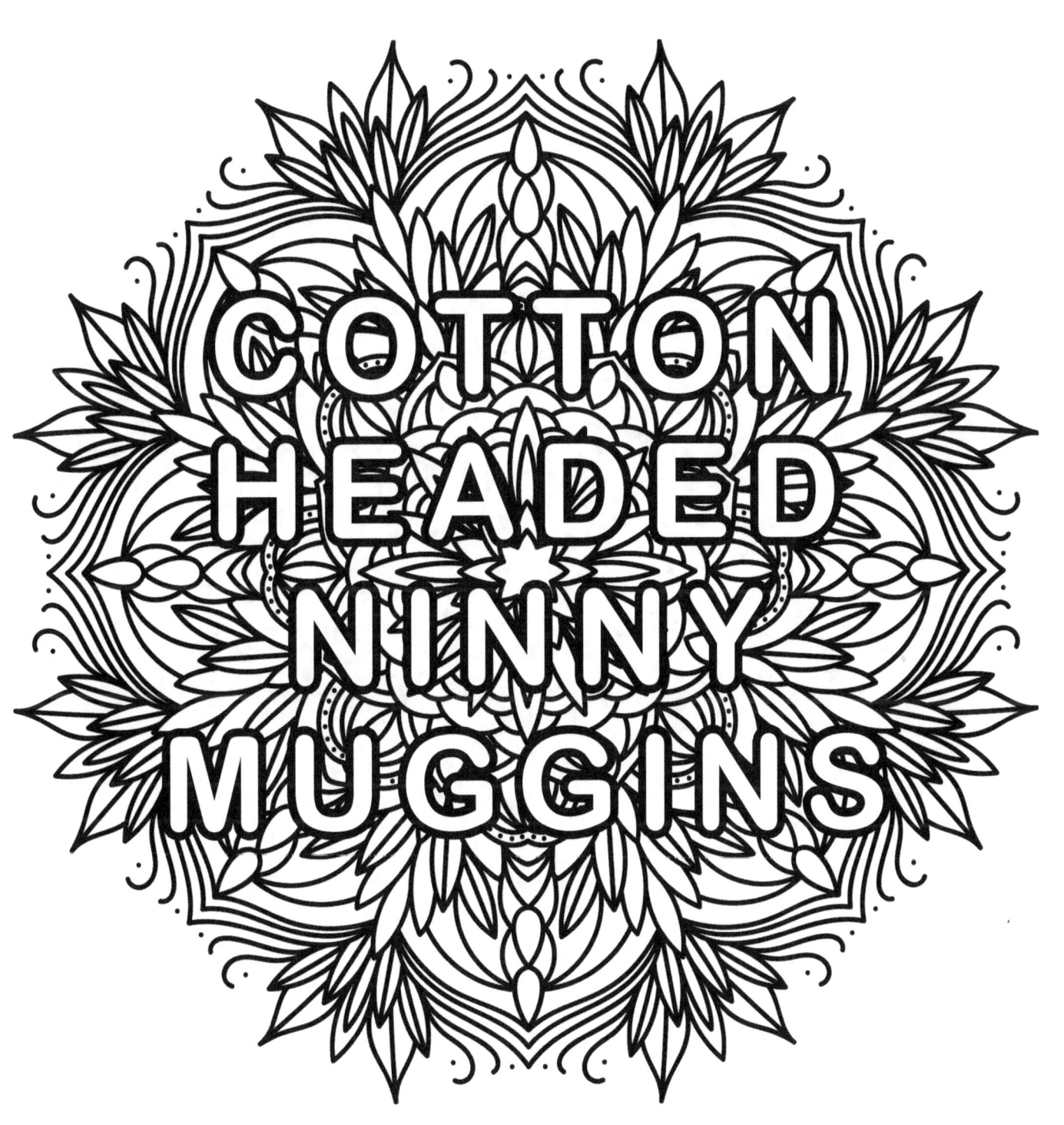

COLORING CREW

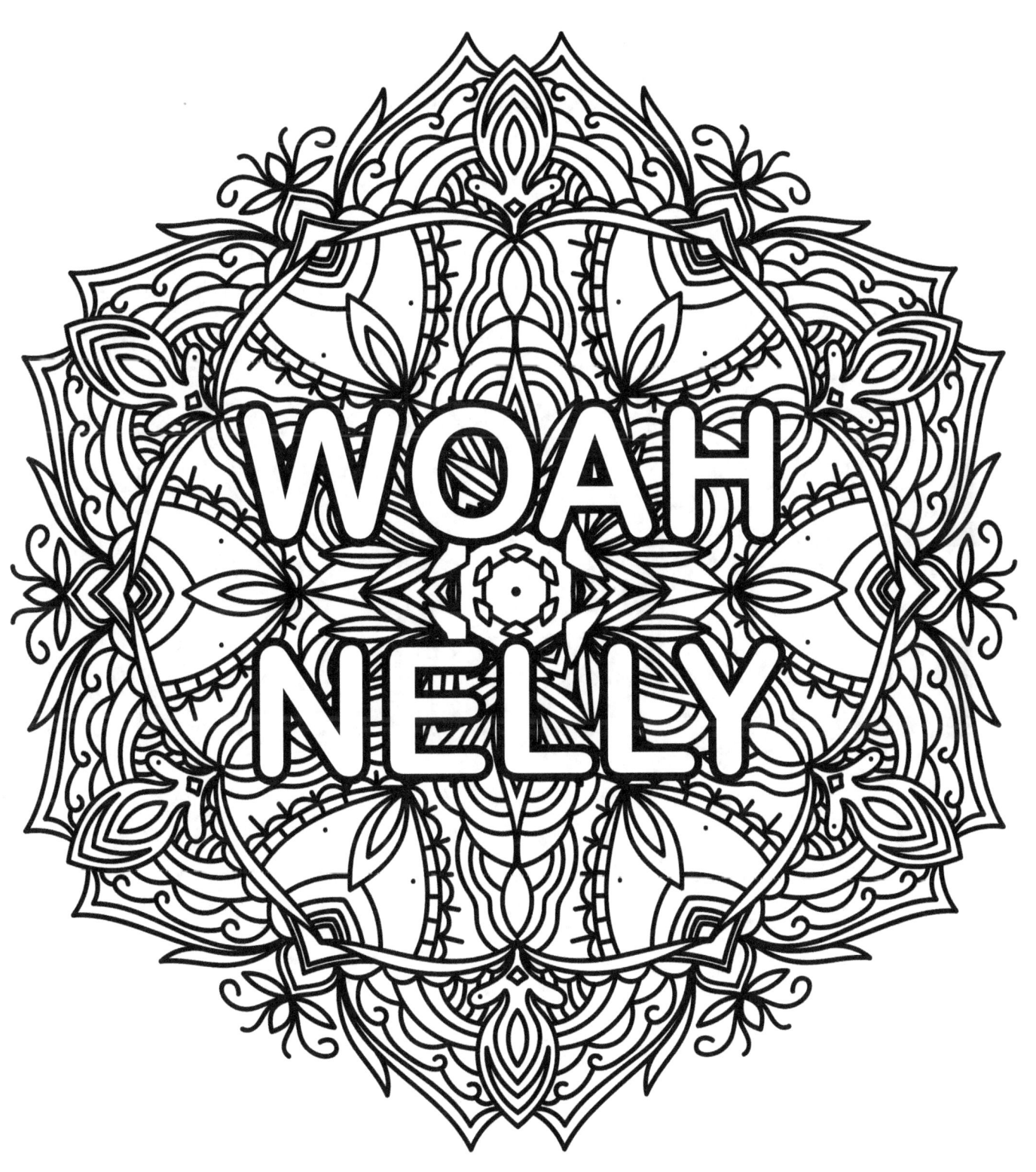

COLORING CREW

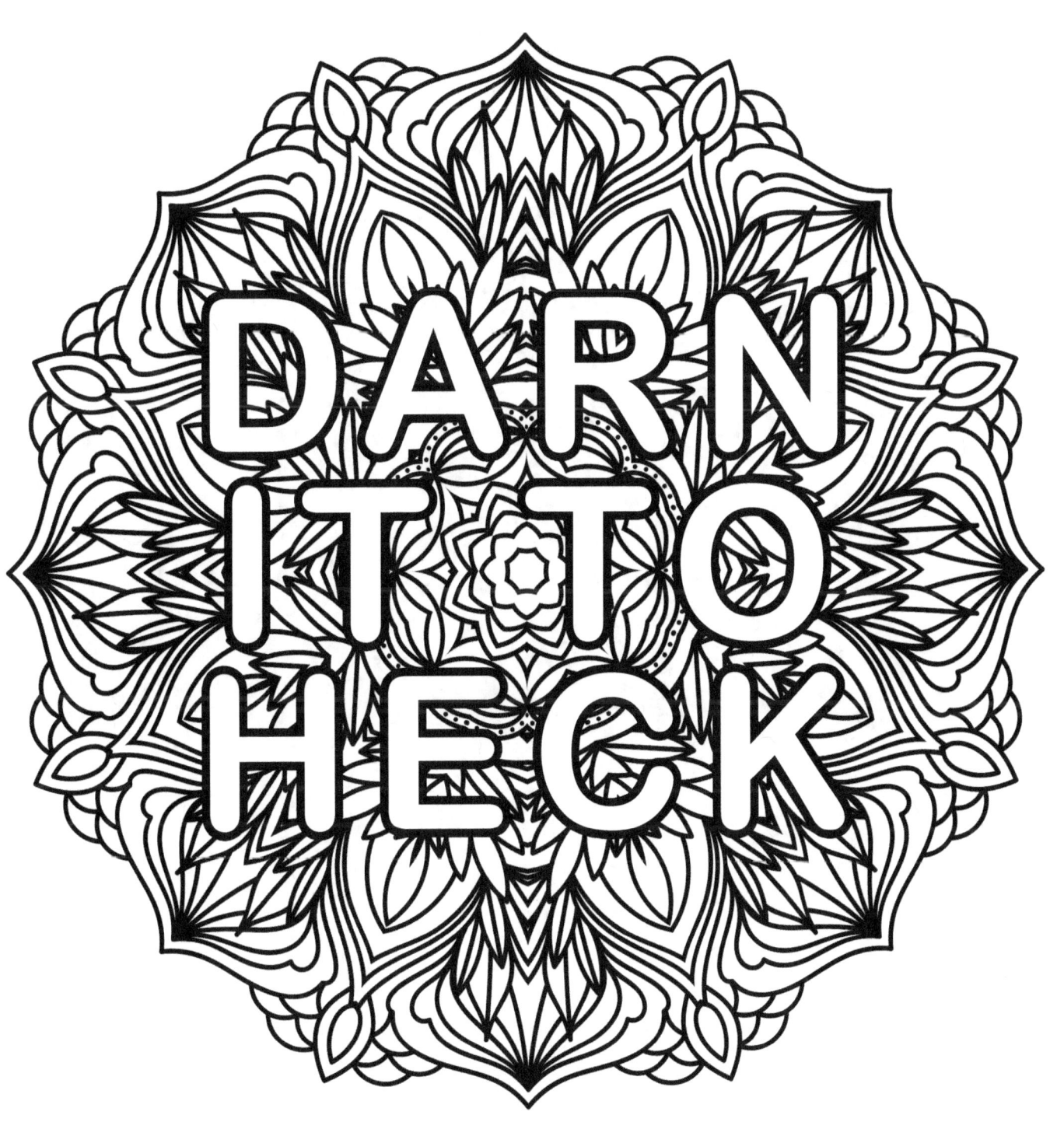

COLORING CREW

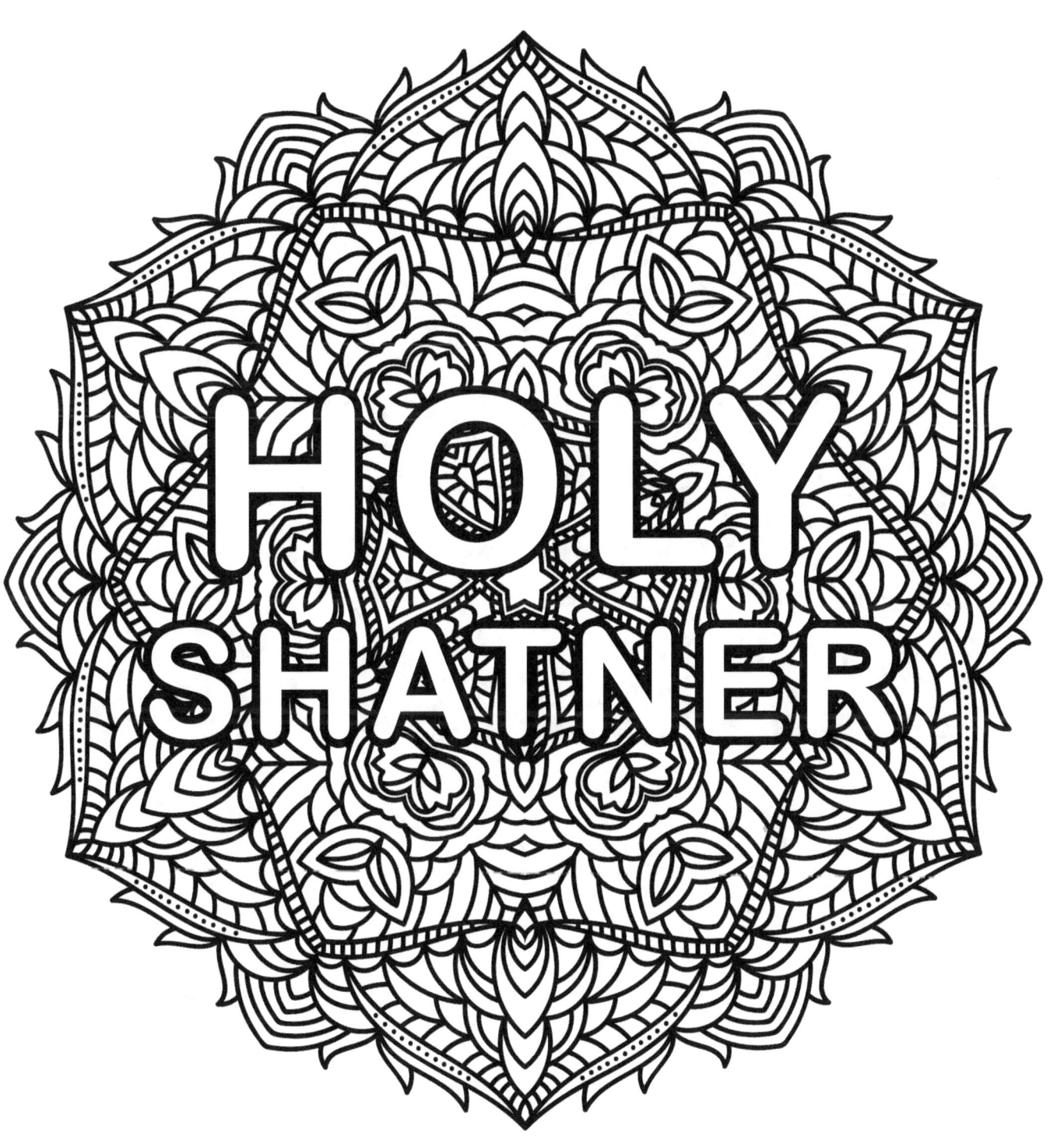

COLORING CREW

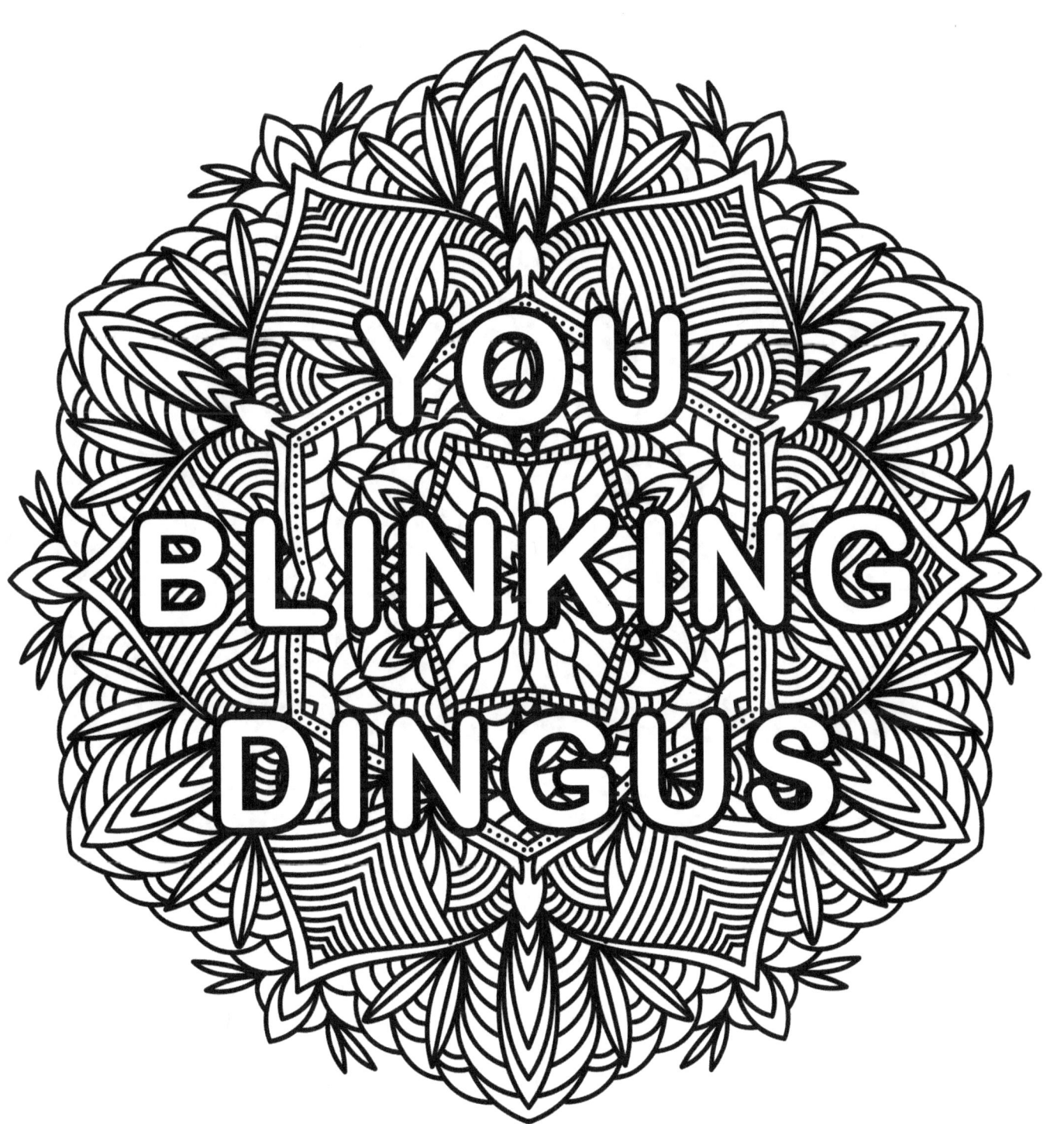

COLORING CREW

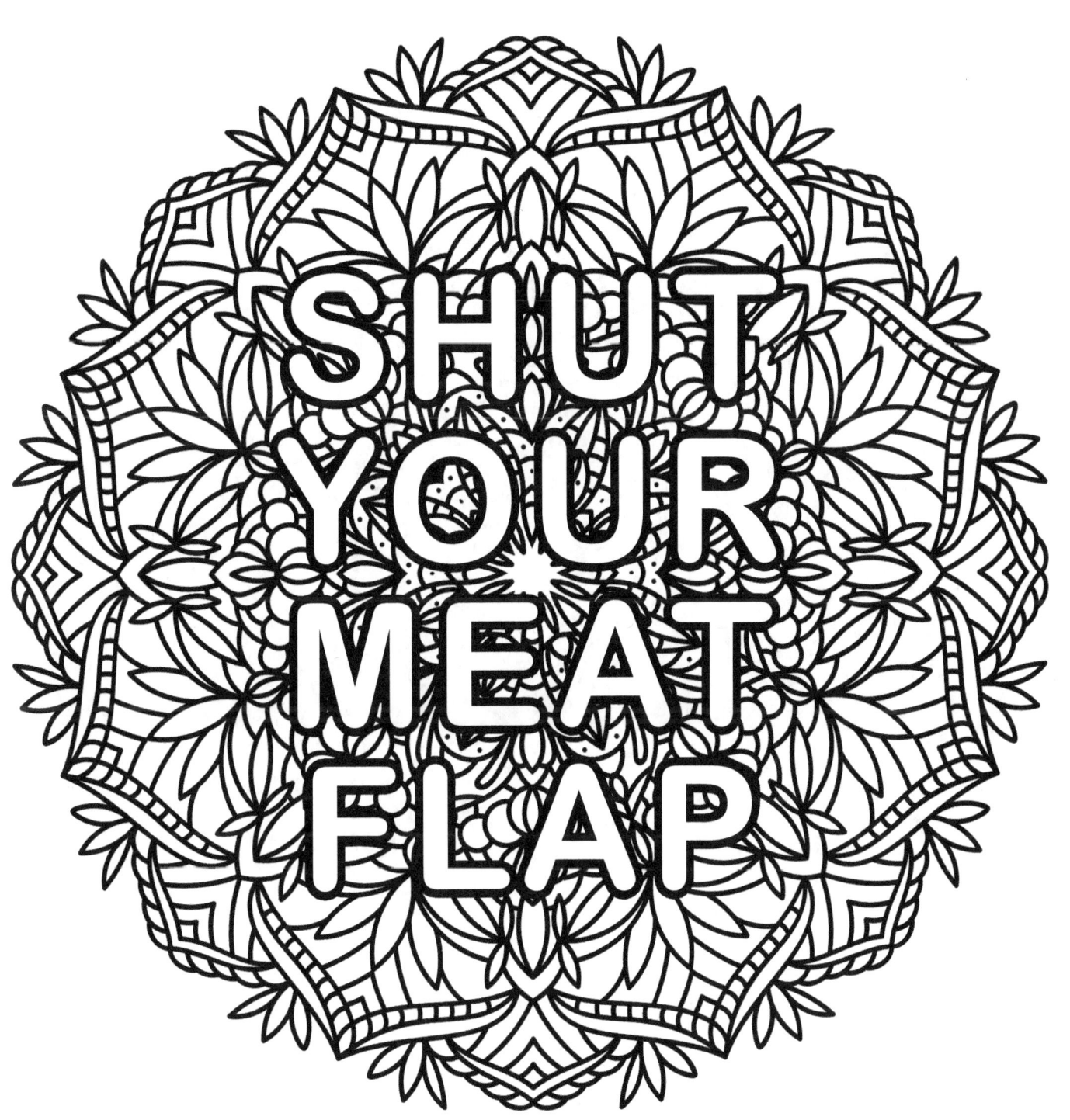

COLORING CREW

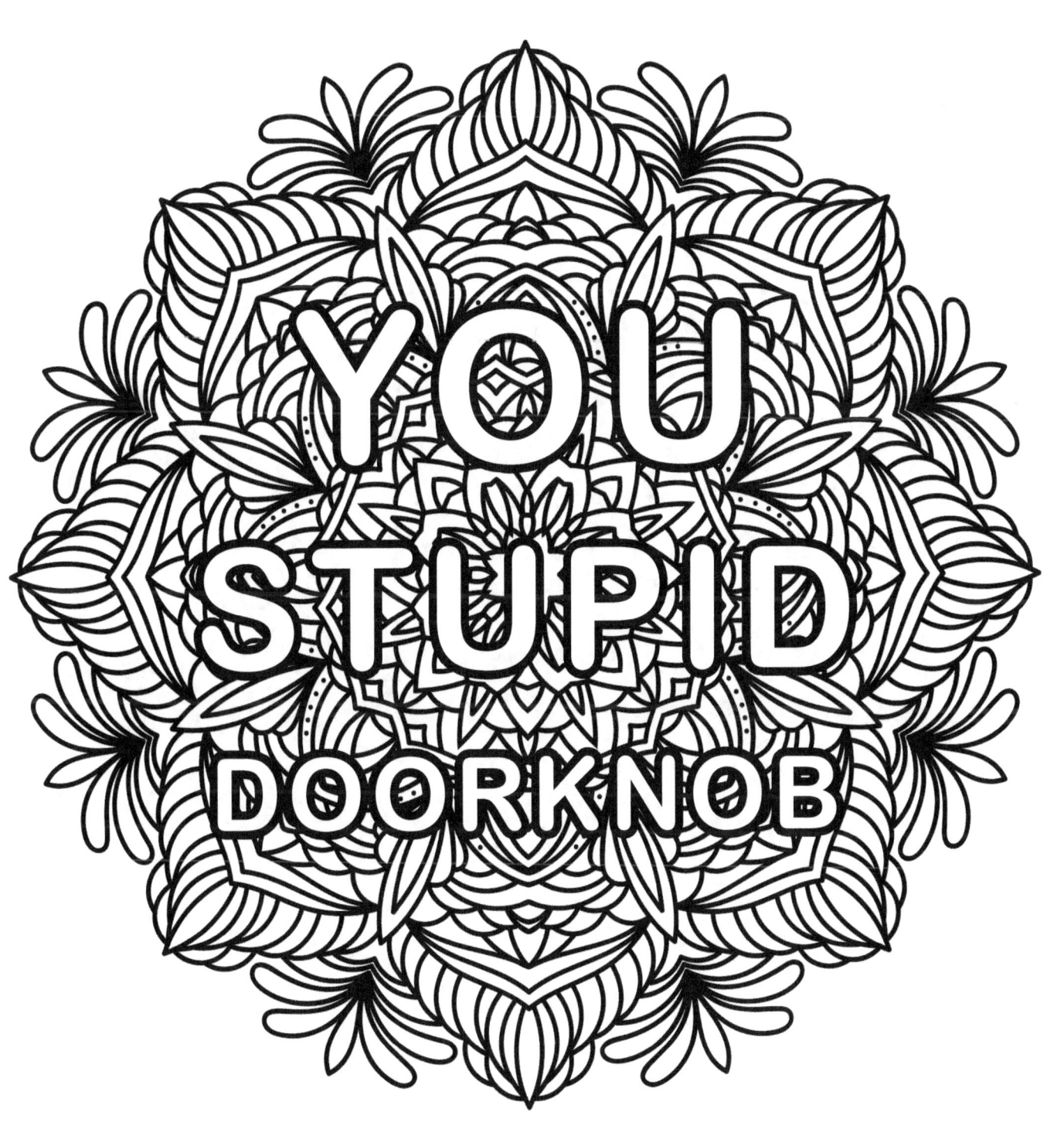

COLORING CREW

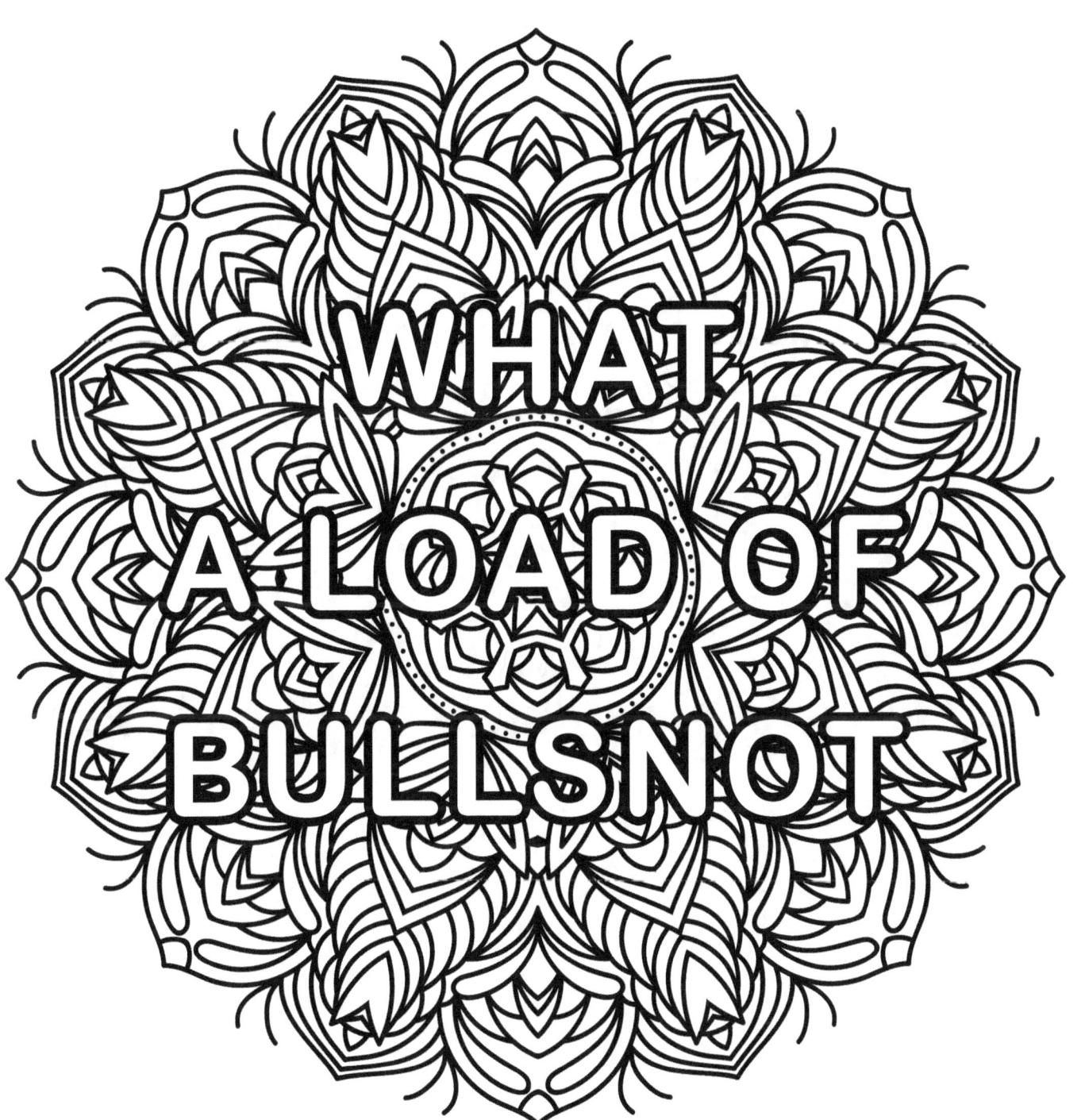

COLORING CREW

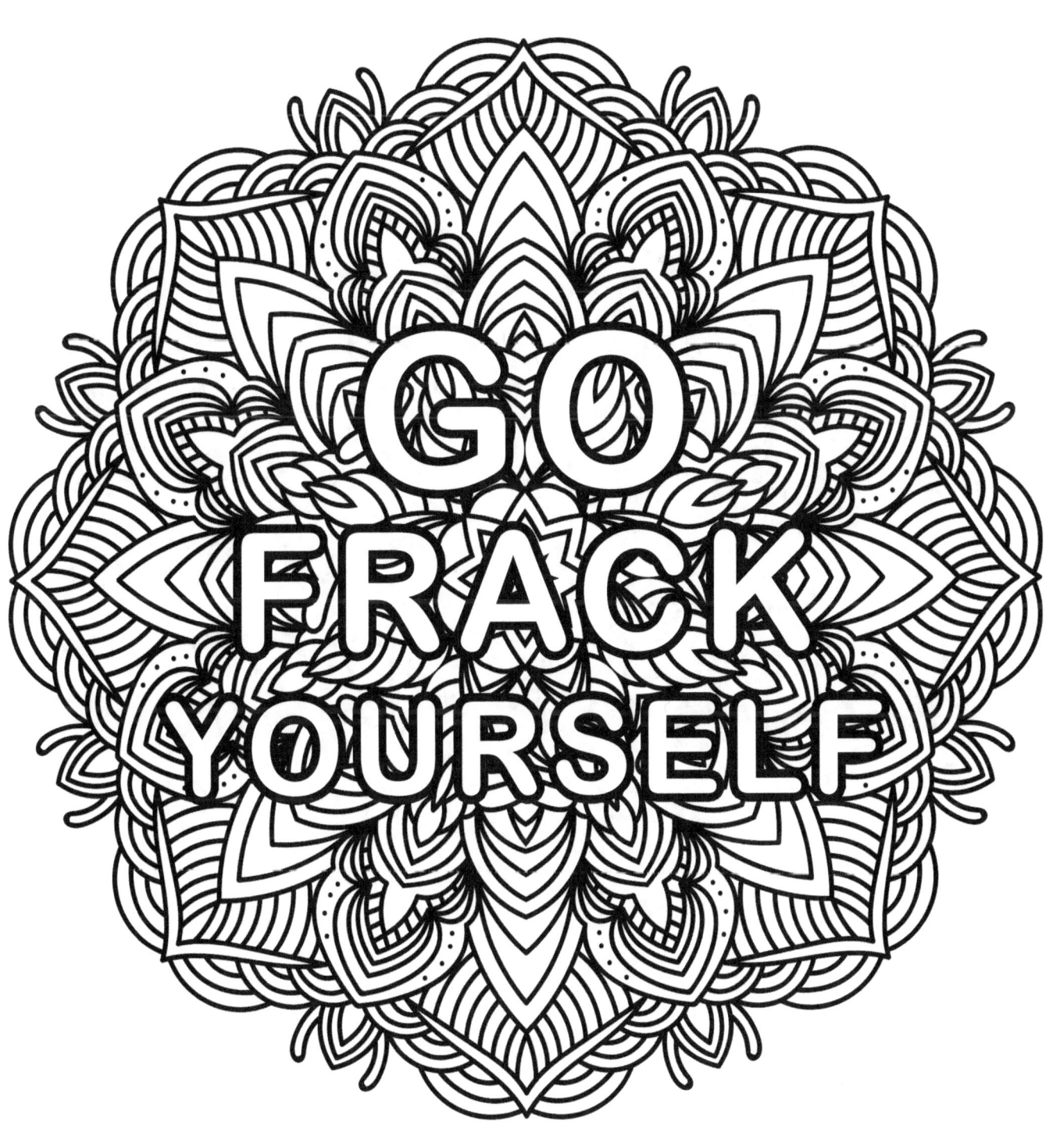

COLORING CREW

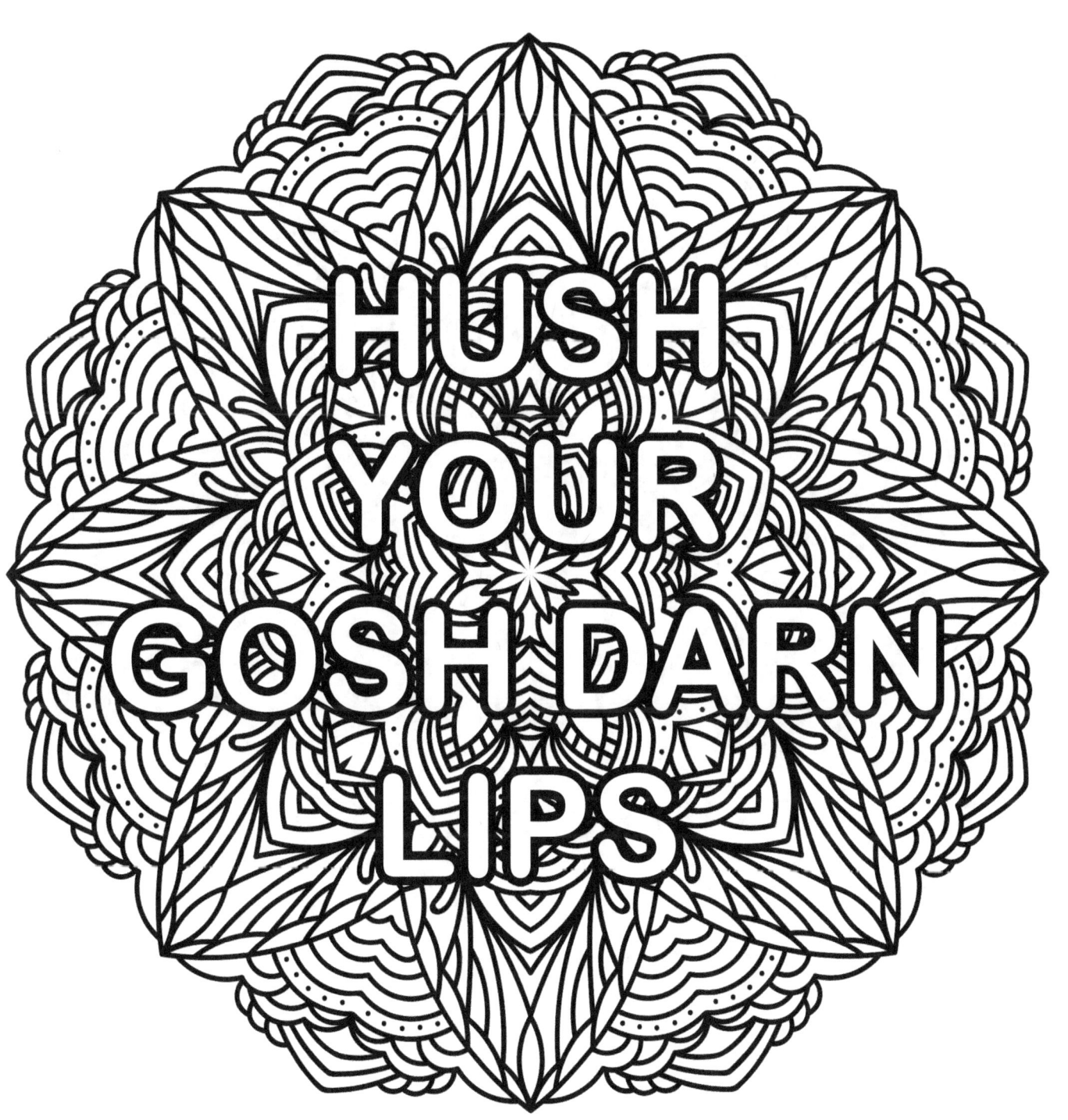

COLORING CREW

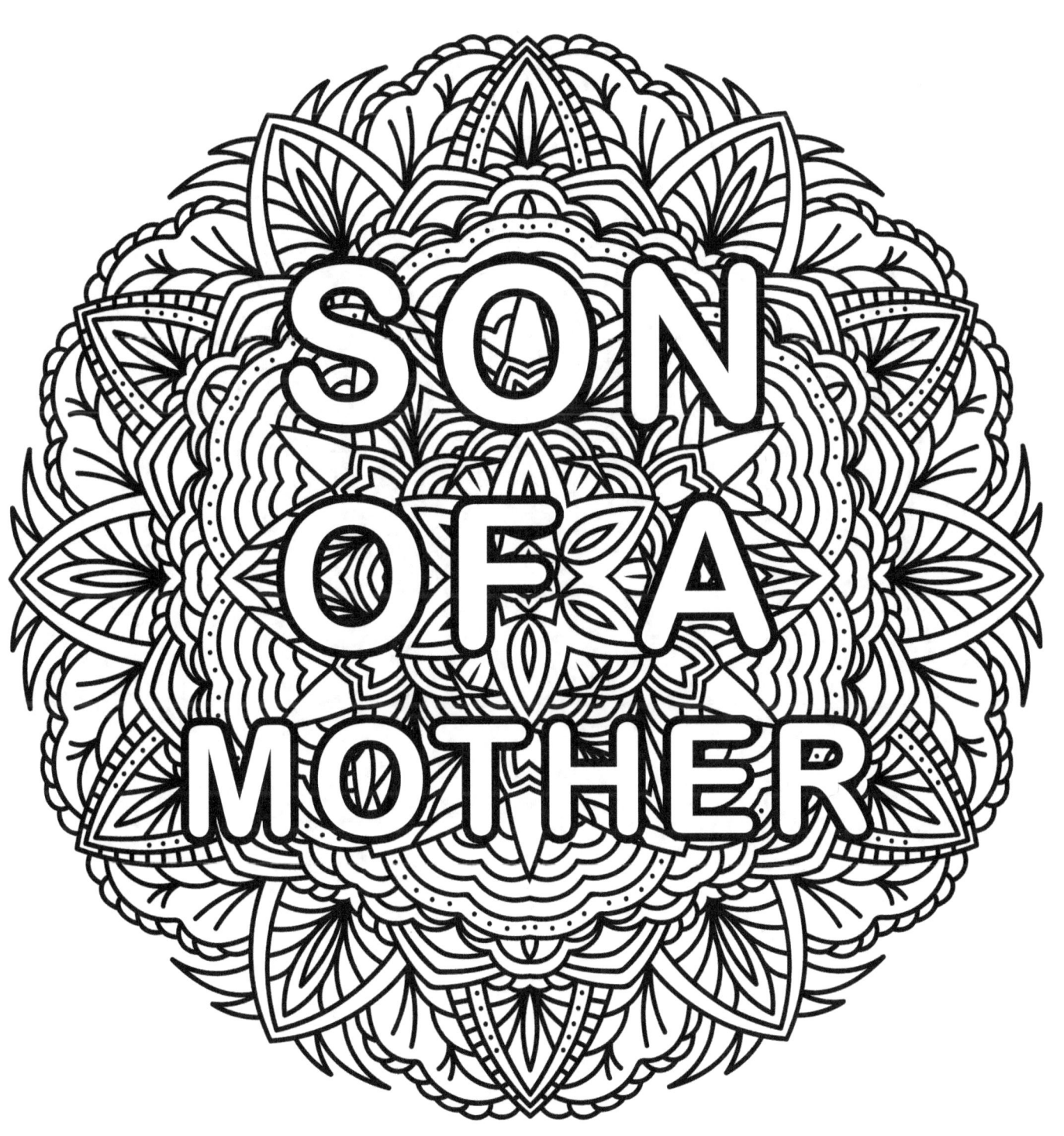

COLORING CREW

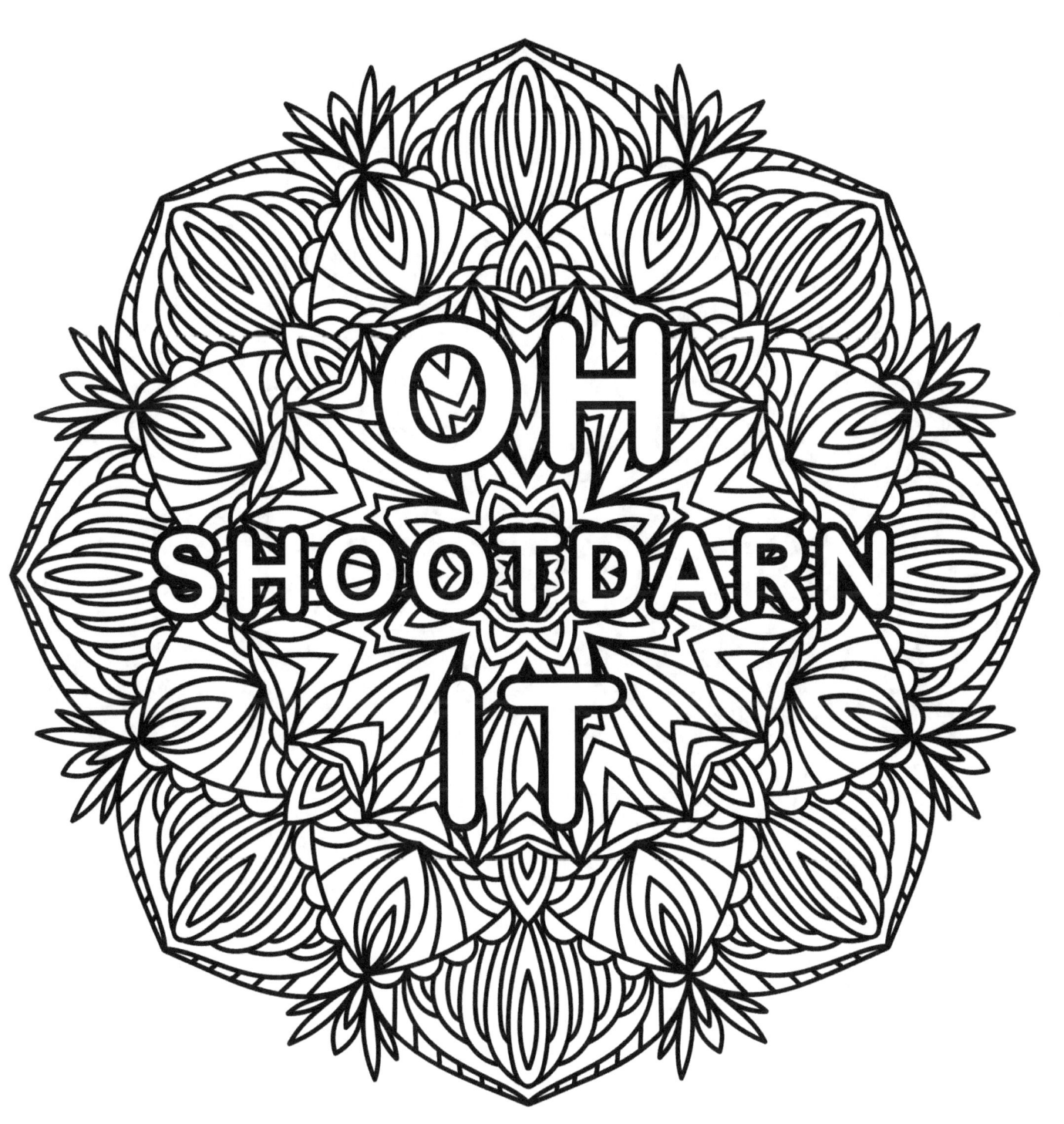

COLORING CREW

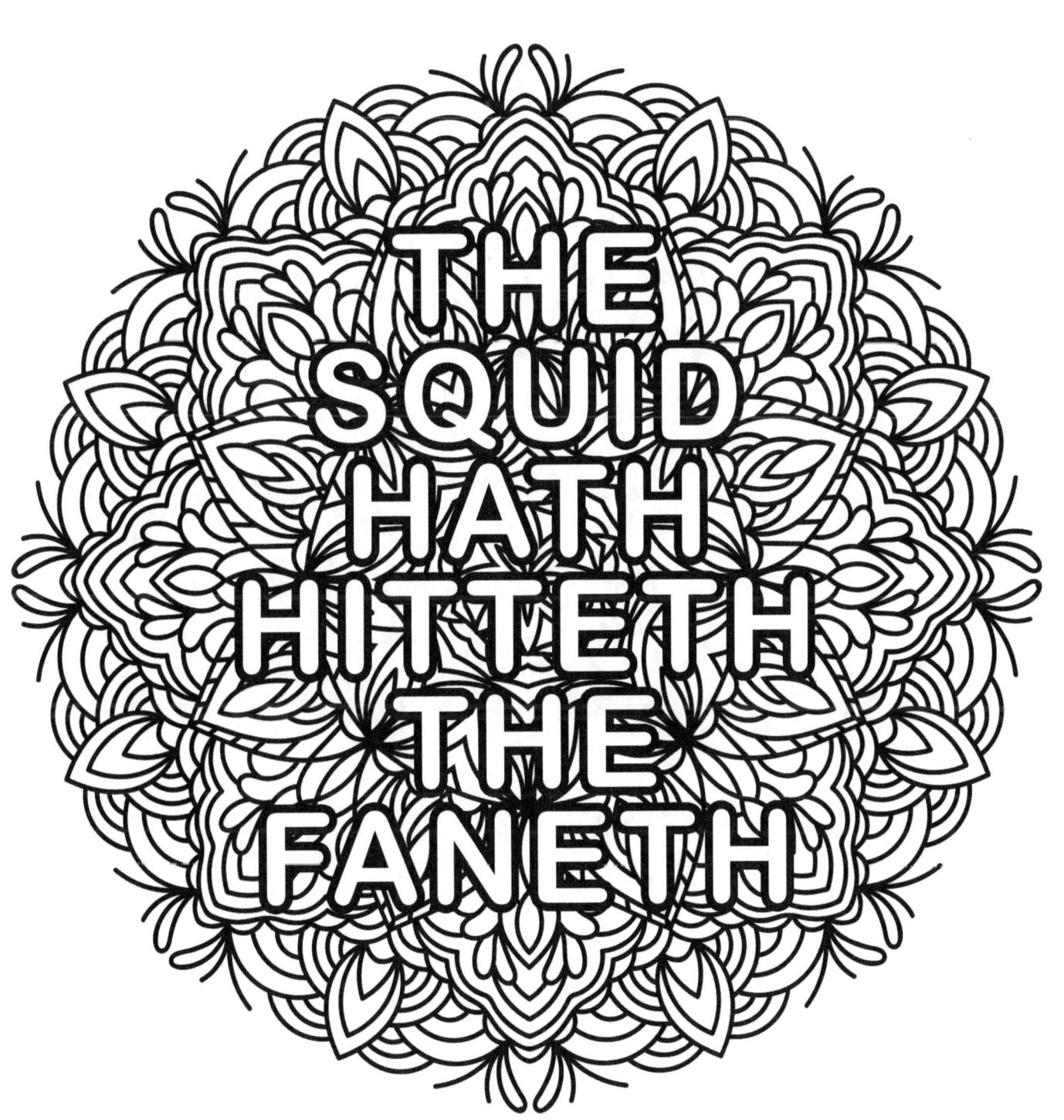

COLORING CREW

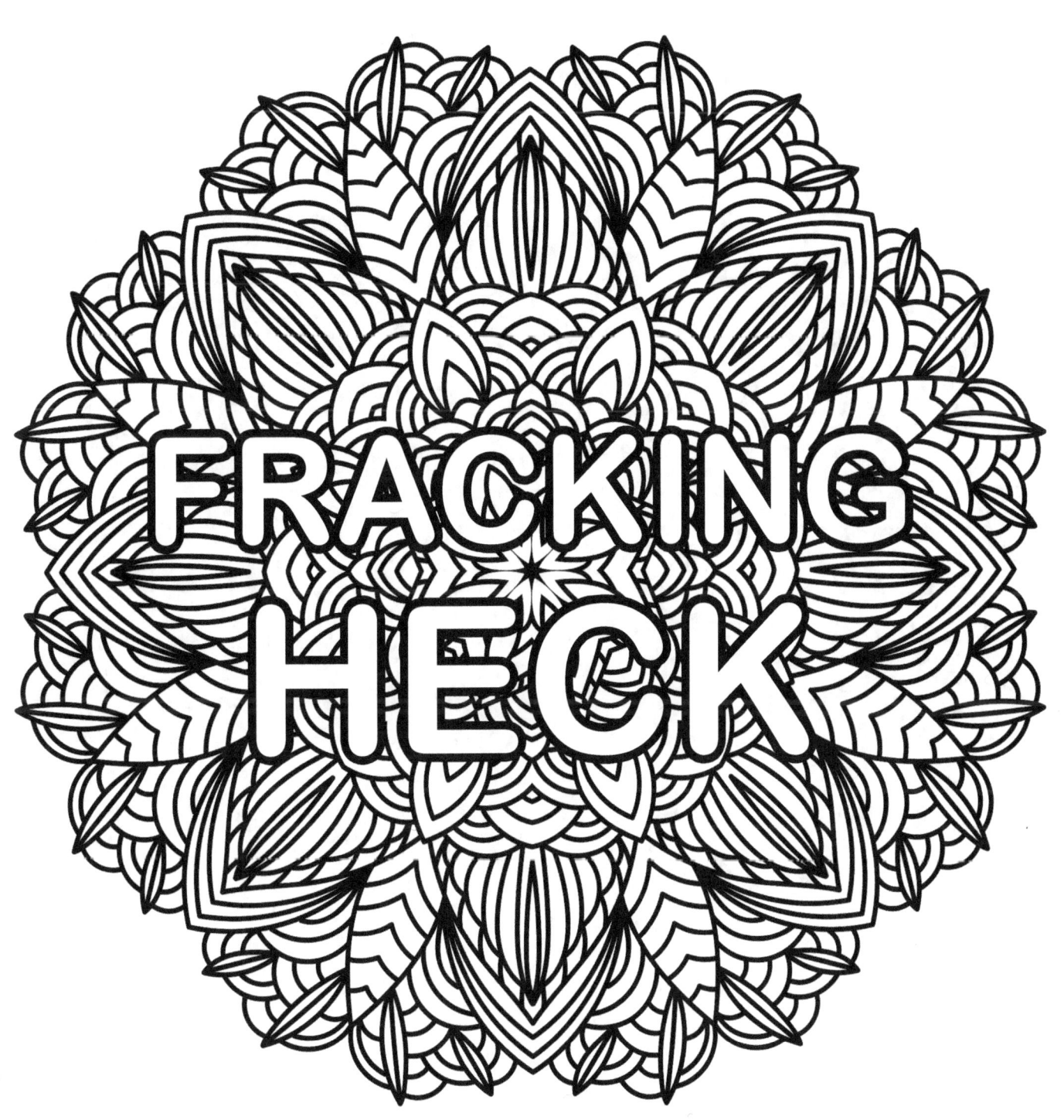

COLORING CREW

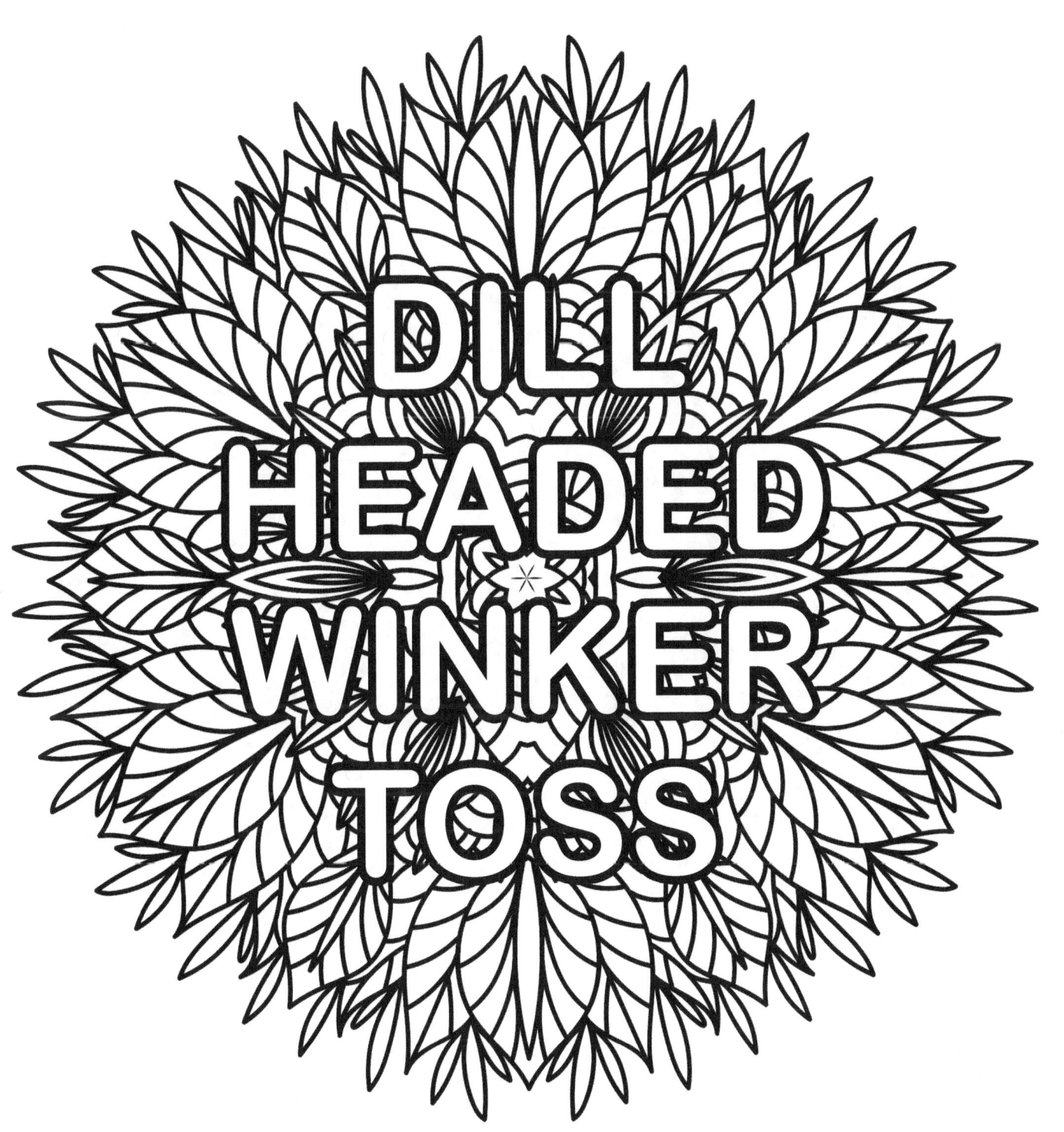

COLORING CREW

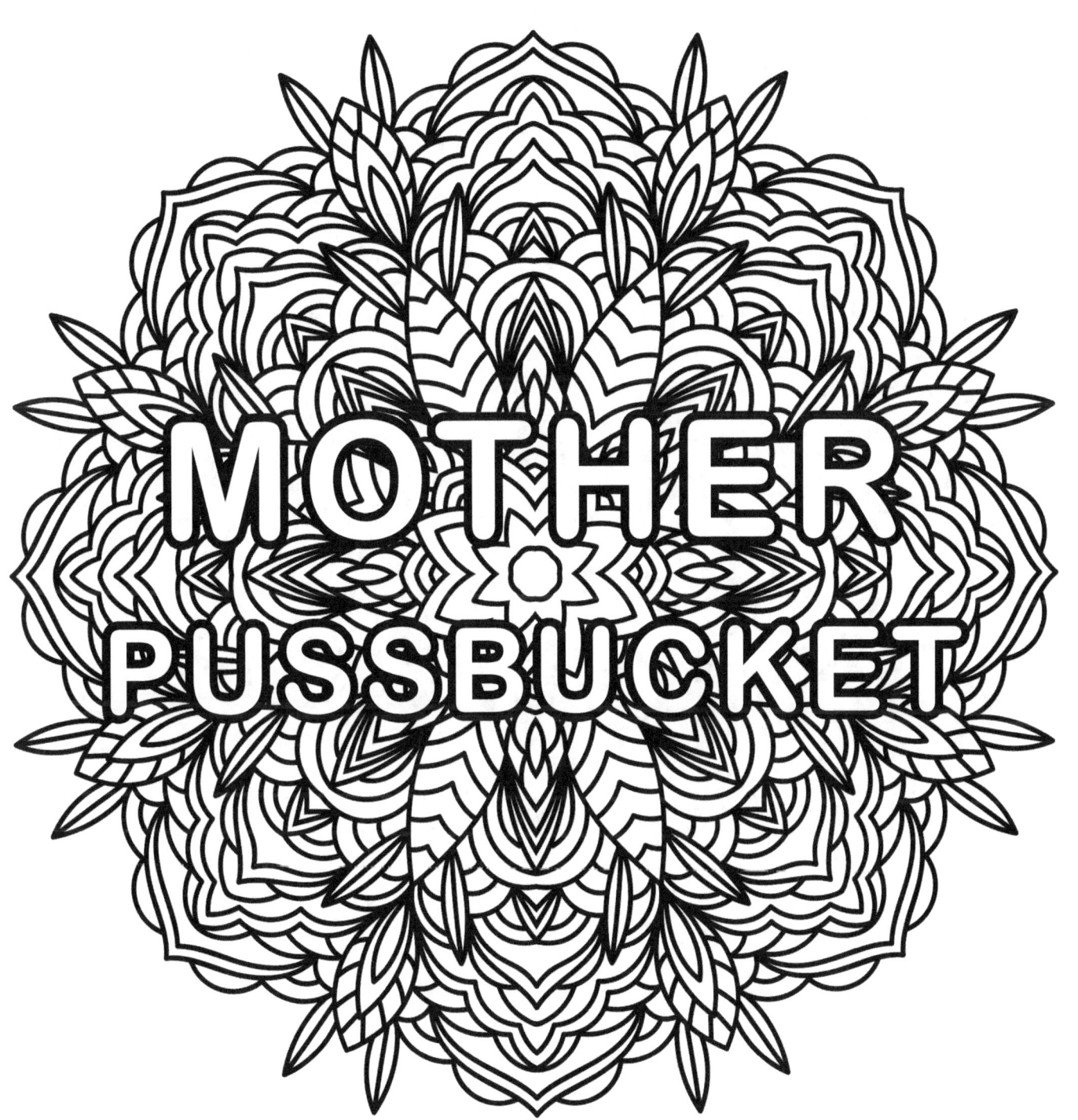

COLORING CREW

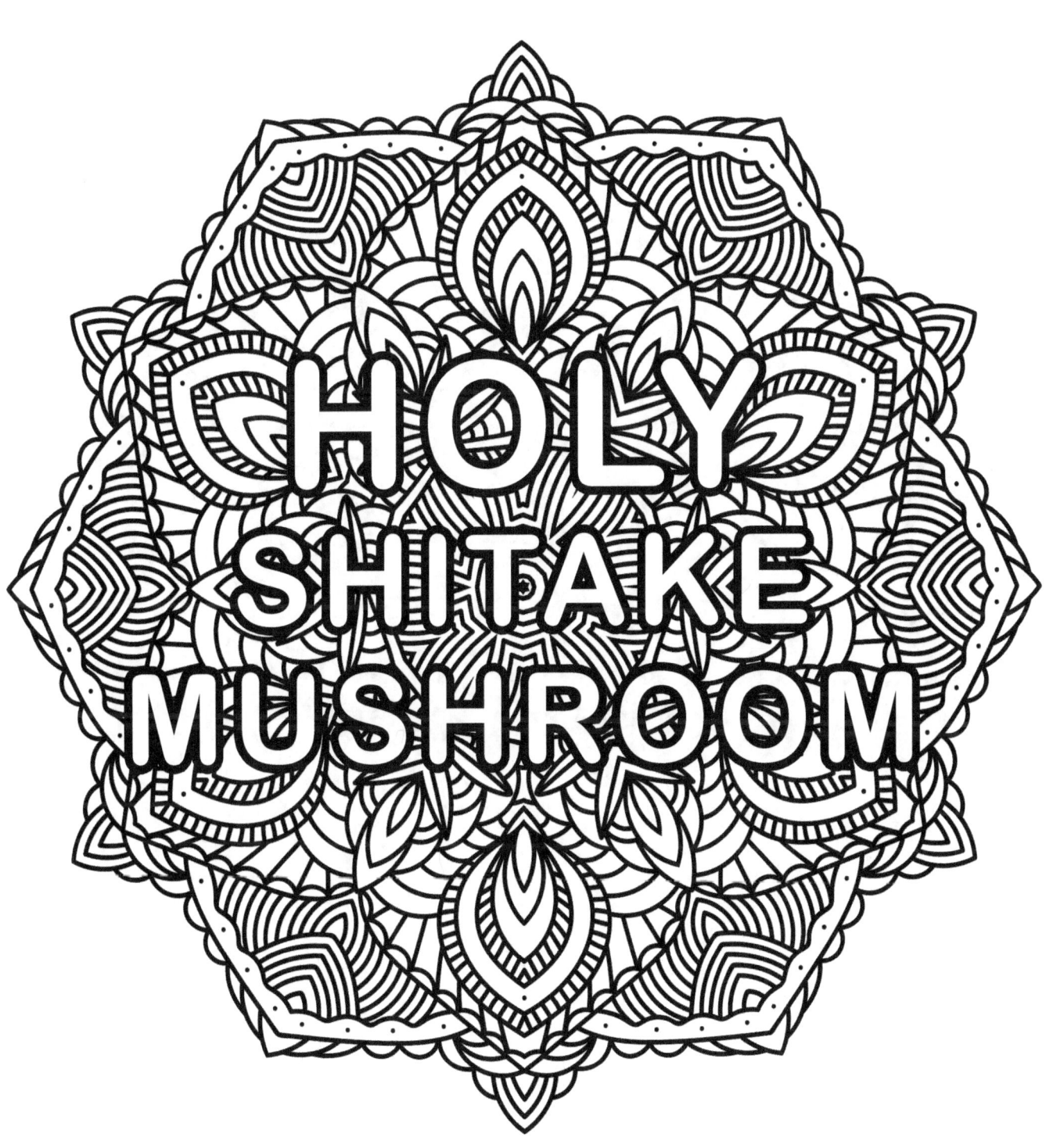

COLORING CREW

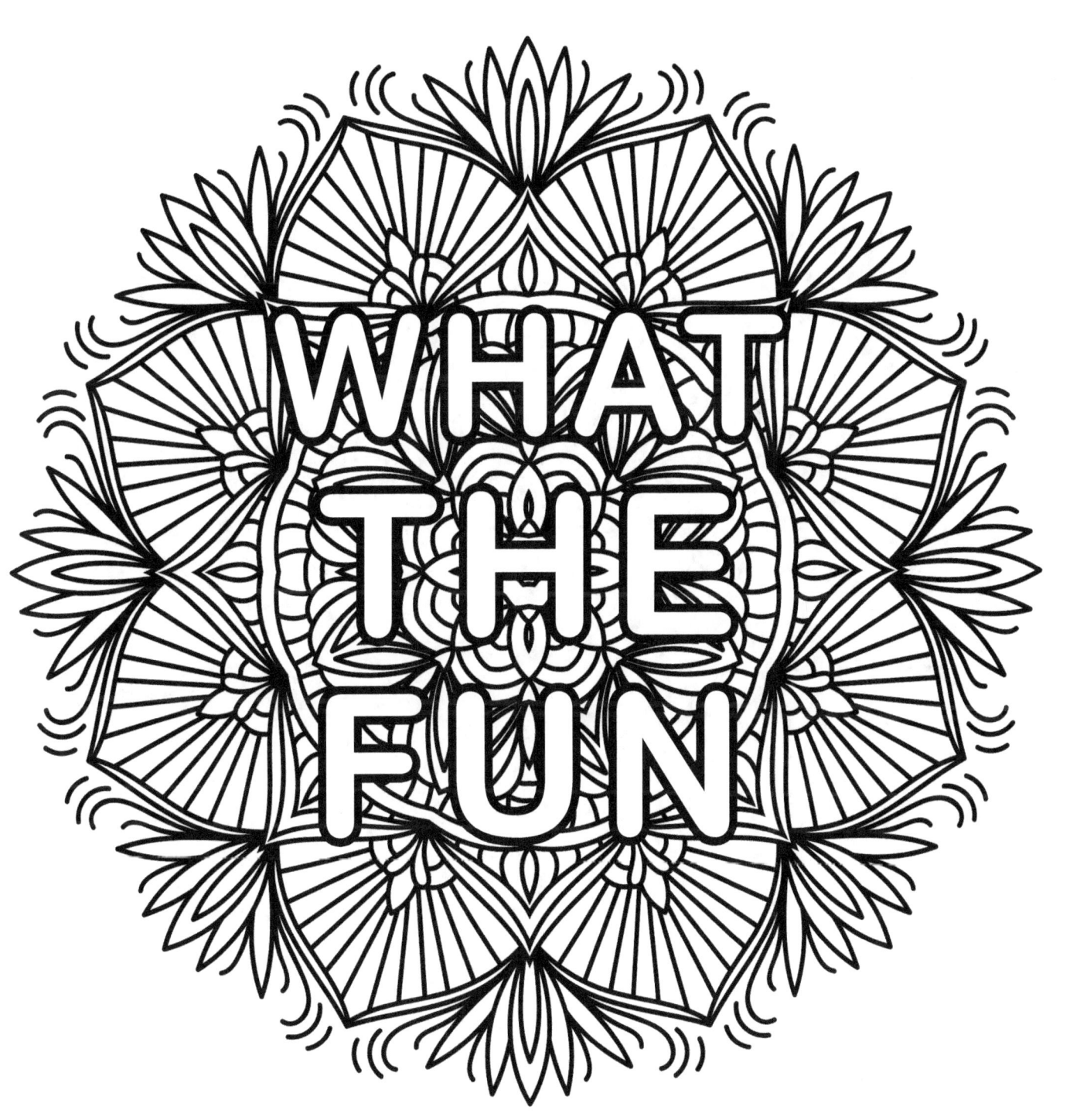

COLORING CREW

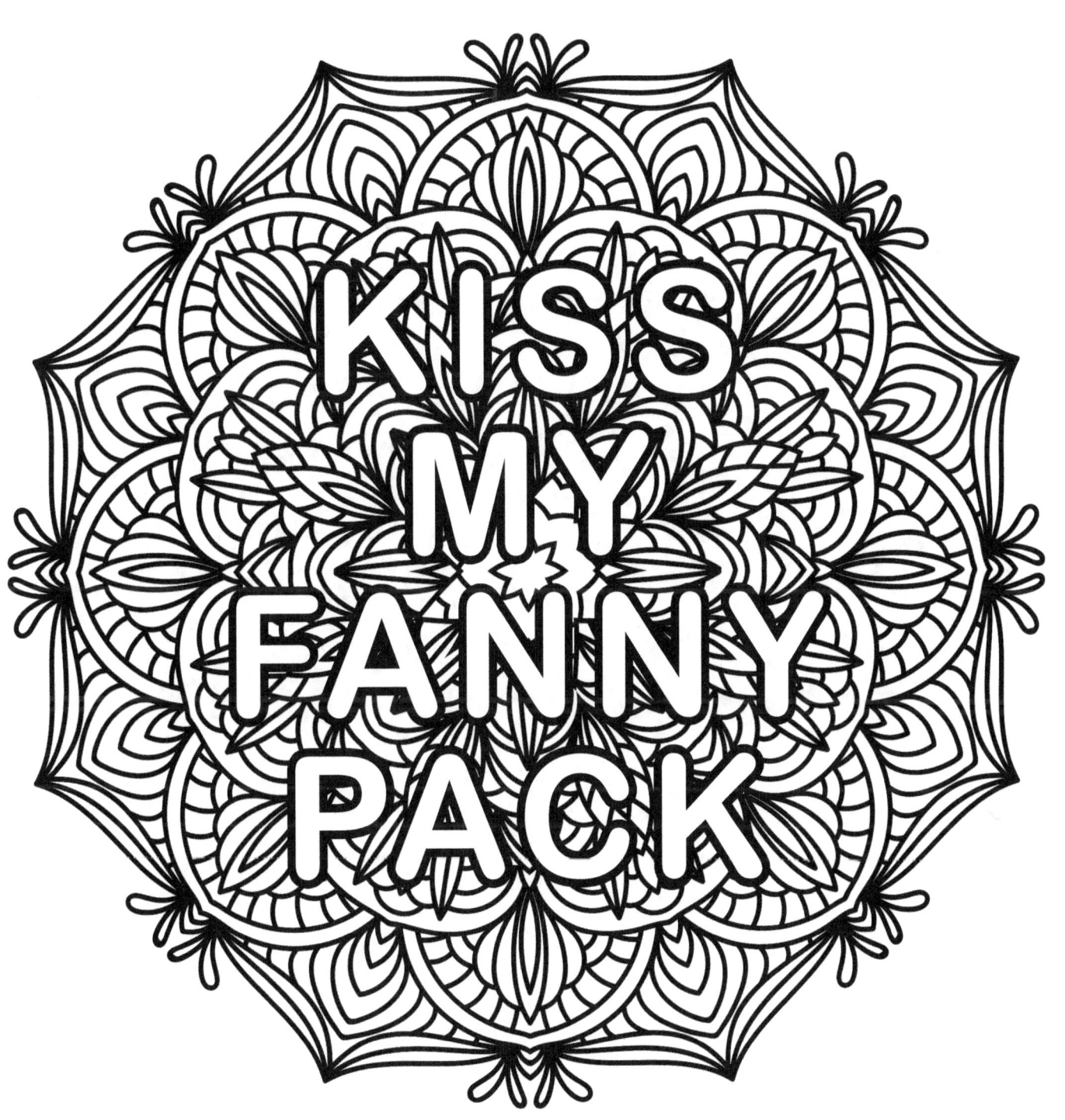

COLORING CREW

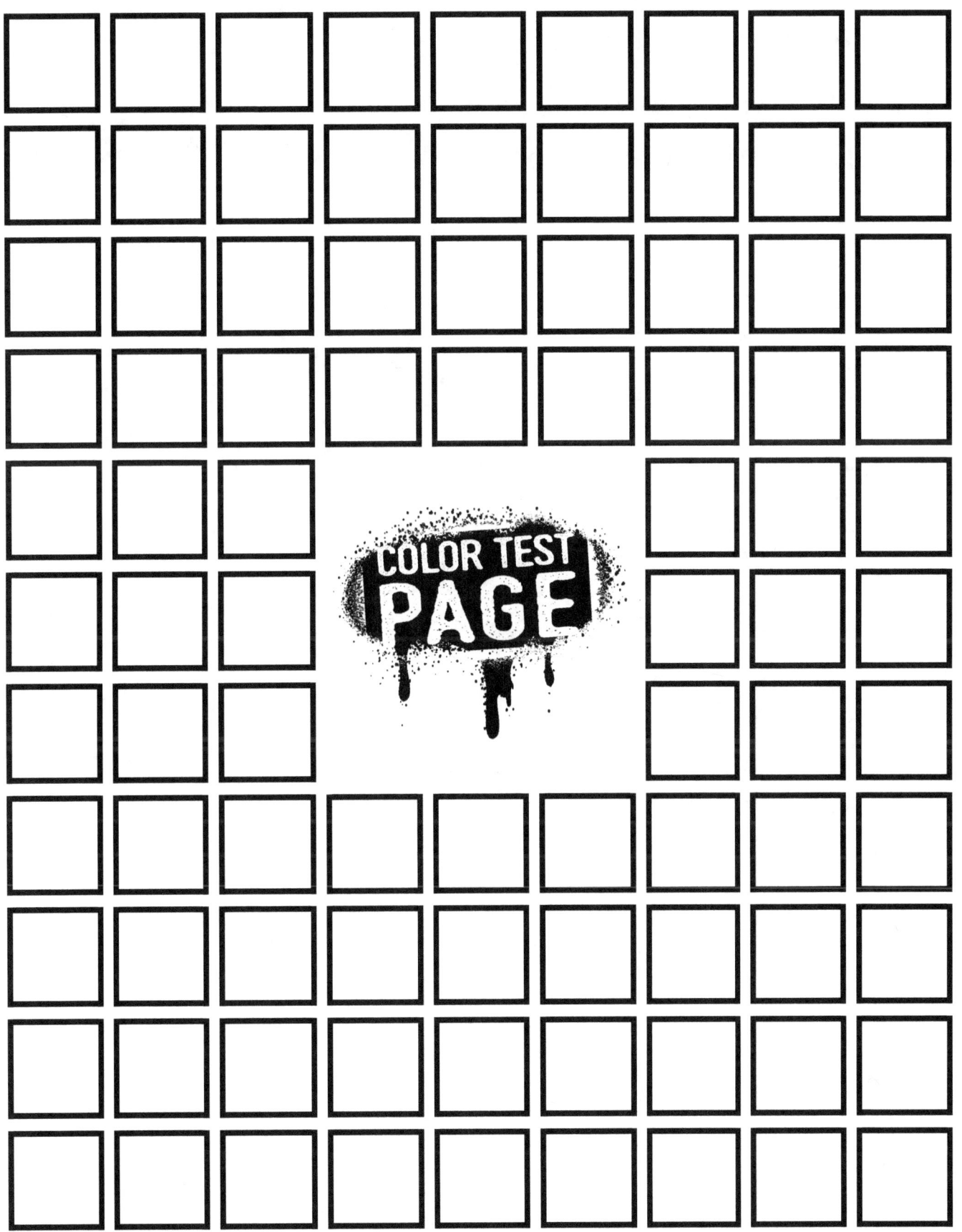

COLORING CREW

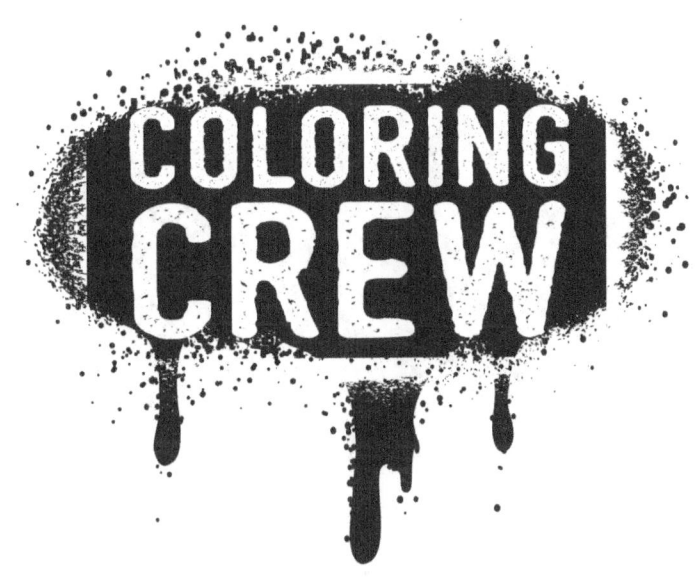

THANKS!
WE HOPE YOU HAD FUN!

IF YOU LIKED THIS BOOK THEN YOU YOU CAN VIEW OUR FULL RANGE OF HILARIOUS ADULT COLORING BOOKS BY GOING TO AMAZON AND SEARCHING FOR "COLORING CREW" AND THEN CLICKING ON OUR AUTHOR PAGE.

THANKS AGAIN!

COLORING CREW

www.ingramcontent.com/pod-product-compliance
Lightning Source LLC
Chambersburg PA
CBHW062125220526
45471CB00010B/3891